Joyful Aging

■   ■   ■

Geri Marr Burdman, Ph.D.

GERIMAR PUBLICATIONS
A Division of Gerimar Educational Services
P.O. Box 357
Mercer Island, WA, 98040
U.S.A.
(206)232-7029

Cover design, book design and graphics:
Jeanne Doran, Bainbridge Island, WA
Editor: Susie Anschell

Library of Congress Catalog Card Number: 90-086008
ISBN: 1-878715-09-7

Cover art based on a woodcut by Aristide Maillol.

Dedicated
to all who seek quality and joy
throughout the life span.

especially
to Barbara + Dick —

Best wishes,

Bob + Geri
Prescott AZ
Aug, 2000

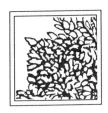

Contents

Life is a full circle, widening until it joins the circle motions of the infinite.

– Anais Nin

This book is about aging healthfully — with meaning, purpose and joy. The circle represents continuity, the cycle of our lives from birth to death.

Entering into the world, we are dependent upon those who care for us. As we grow and our world expands, we realize our own potential and experience a process whereby the mystery of life is slowly revealed to us.

Each stage of life is a stepping stone in preparation for the next. The journey is a continuous one. Our choices and attitudes create our reality all along the way.

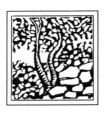

*Creating
Purpose
and Meaning
in Aging*

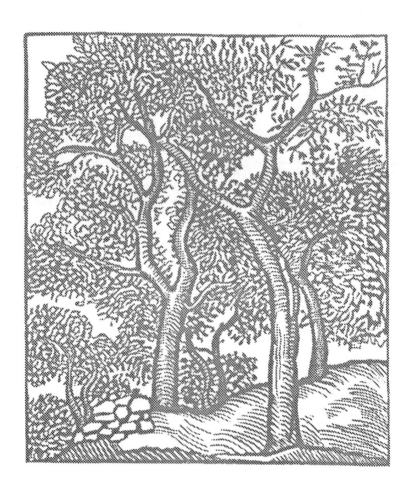

Friendship is a sheltering tree . . .
　　　　　　　　　　– S. Coleridge

You might meaningfully speak of
an Art of Aging . . .

– Erich Fromm

Until Joan and Erik Erikson's work on adult development several decades ago, the major focus in the study of human development was early childhood and adolescence. The light they shed on later adulthood has been a critical factor in enhancing our understanding of the human life cycle.

Stages of Development

We all face challenges at every stage of growth and development. Our ability to become healthy and whole is dependent upon the manner in which we deal with these challenges. The strength derived at each stage provides a stepping stone for the next and the process goes on from birth to death.

Infancy

This is the stage at which hope and faith and basic trust are developed. As our world expands, this trust grows, nurtured by the quality and sensitivity of the care we receive. It is during this stage that we derive the potential for confidence in other humans and faith in the future.

Early Childhood

At this stage, willpower is developed and through it the capacity to act independently. This is a decisive age for the development of the potential for love, cooperation and freedom of self-expression. This stage forms the basis for independence and self-reliance later in life.

Pre-School Age

The objective at this stage is to achieve a sense of purpose—the courage to envision and pursue goals in life, uninhibited by fears.

We have a surplus of energy at this age and we forget failures easily, proceeding with growing confidence and judgment. It is during this period that we learn quickly about sharing and making things cooperatively with other children as well as adults.

School Age

The goal of this stage is a sense of competency. The major events revolve around entrance into school life. As children, we are sometimes forced to forget past wishes and hopes, and our imaginations are tamed by school work. We begin to produce things and to apply ourselves to given skills and tasks.

Adolescence

Childhood ends and youth begins; there is rapid body growth and genital maturity. We seek a sense of *identity* — a confidence that the inner sameness and continuity achieved in the preceding stages are now matched by the way others view us.

At this stage peer acceptance and career goals become all-important to our sense of well-being.

Young Adulthood

After the struggle for identity, the young adult generally seeks relationships of intimacy, mutual trust, and respect. This intimacy should not mean a loss of self-identity or individuality but rather an extension of it.

Midlife

Midlife is often a time of re-evaluation of our goals and life events as we confront once again the deep need for a sense of identity and purpose. This period can be equally painful and challenging as adolescence and earlier stages. It is often a time of intense concern about the effects of our life events on ourselves and others, now and in the future.

Later Life

This stage calls for acceptance and consolidation of our life course. The supreme goal is *wisdom* and a sense of peace with ourselves in the larger scheme of things.

Old age can be a satisfying and emotionally healthy time of life, a time of potential growth and self-enhancement. Later life should be recognized as a developmental stage equal in importance to the younger years. As we age, we continue to be worthy of self-development; we must give greater emphasis to that SELF.

■　　■　　■

We all have capacities, talents directions, missions, callings . . .
The task is, if we are willing to take it seriously, to help ourselves to be all that we are in potentiality.

– Maslow

Abraham Maslow's well-known Hierarchy of Needs speaks to our human universal longing for self-actualization and self development throughout the life span.

Maslow's Hierarchy of Needs

Physiological needs.

The most basic, most powerful, most obvious of all needs are those for physical survival: food, water, air, shelter, and sleep. Until a person has satisfied these needs, all others will be pushed into the background.

Safety needs.

Once the physiological needs are sufficiently satisfied, *safety needs* emerge. Not only physical safety but also consistency, fairness, and a certain amount of routine in daily living are important.

Belongingness and love needs.

Once the physiological and safety needs are met, needs for love, affection and belongingness emerge. We seek positive relations with others in order to satisfy the universal human need to be deeply understood and accepted.

Esteem needs.

Most of us have two types of esteem needs: self-respect and esteem from others. Esteem needs result from a desire for confidence, competence, mastery, adequacy, achievement, independence, and freedom.

Self-actualization needs.

Self-actualization is basic to human motivation. What we can be, we must become. There is a need for continuous development of our potential. The need for self-actualization generally emerges after a reasonable satisfaction of the love and esteem needs.

Desire to know and understand.

A characteristic of good mental health is curiosity and immersion in something worthy of our efforts — a search for deep personal meaning.

Aesthetic needs.

The need for and appreciation of beauty is almost universally present and profoundly experienced in healthy, self-actualizing people.

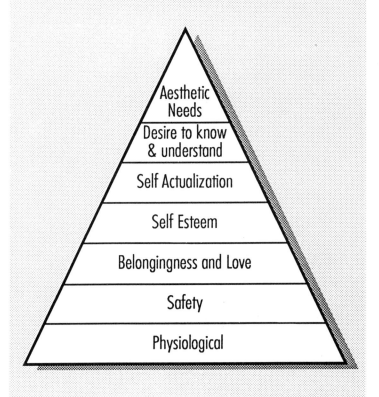

Maslow's
Hierarchy of Needs

We are all travelers — from birth to death — travelling between eternities.
                                    – Anon

■   ■   ■

When you find out who you really are, it is beautiful beyond your dreams.
                                    –Sujata

■   ■   ■

The main thing in life is not to be afraid of being human.
                                    – Pablo Casals

Search for Meaning

The search for meaning is a primary motivational factor in humans the world over.

People who seem to be the happiest and healthiest at any age are those who are connected with others by mutual need and a sense of identity. They are active and engaged in life and generally share some common charactaristics:

- an acceptance of responsibility for self and the ability to formulate realistic goals

- a realistic sense of and respect for self

- flexibility and resilience and the capacity to accept joy as well as sorrow

- trust in other human beings and the expectation that this is a reciprocal process

- an ability to give love and to consider the interests of others

- an ability to receive love

- a sense of community and responsibility toward neighbors and fellow humans

- an understanding of the cycle of life

- an acceptance of death as a stage of life.

Life is what our thoughts make it. . .

–Marcus Aurelius

Meaning in life can be discovered:
- *By doing a deed*
- *By experiencing a value*
- *Through suffering*

What matters — above all — is the attitude we take — how we accept life's circumstances.

– Viktor Frankl

Sometimes life's shadows are caused by our standing in our own sunshine.

– Emerson

*We must never forget that we may
also find meaning in life even when
confronted with a hopeless situation,
when facing a fate that cannot be
changed.
When we are no longer able to change
a situation — we are challenged to
change ourselves.*

—Viktor Frankl

*At the core of your being is a positive
and purposeful source from where you
create your reality.*

— Gerimar

The Role of Life Review

All too often the tendency to reminisce about the past has been dismissed as irrelevant. Life review is a universal and normal developmental process. Our memories are quarries of recollections that we can mine at will. The process of reviewing past experiences provides an opportunity for integrating the past as well as a linking with our present and with our future selves.

For some this review may provide new dimensions and a sense of place; for others it may serve as a catalyst for inner healing. Emotions vary in the process, but there nearly always is an element of pain to work through as old unresolved issues surface and are addressed.

What lies behind us and what lies before us are tiny matters compared to what lies within us.

—*Emerson*

*Life's fulfillment finds constant
contradiction in its path, but this is
necessary for the sake of its advance.*

– Tagore

Life Review Experience

Go deep within yourself and look at *your* personal journey and search for meaning. What do you see? What are the pluses? What are the minuses? What are the key events in your life that make you who you are today? Where do you want to be? Can you create that reality? How?

On the following page, draw or write your feelings about each stage of life you have experienced—or expect to experience—from birth to death.

*Be open — listen deep within
yourself . . . the answers will come.*

Personal life review notes:

As the cells in my body renew
And my purpose in life I review
I find, growing older
I'm now growing bolder
And increasingly hard to subdue!

— *Helen Green Ansley*

Be patient toward all that is unsolved
in your heart and try to love the
questions themselves . . .

— *Rainer Maria Rilke*

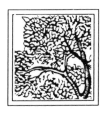

*Health
Promotion
and Aging*

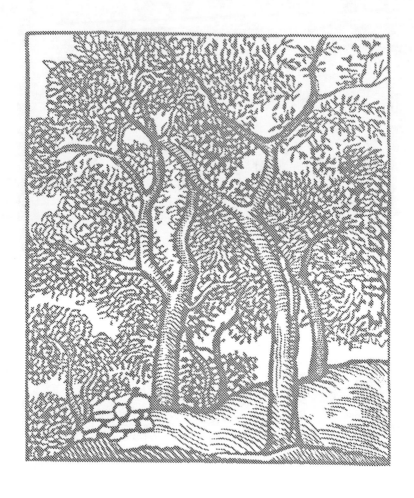

As the twig is bent, so the tree inclines . . .

— *Virgil*

In the long run we shape our lives and we shape ourselves. The process never ends...And the choices we make are ultimately our own responsibility.   – *Eleanor Roosevelt*

■   ■   ■

The dynamic nature of health is reflected in the World Health Organization's definition:

Health is a state of physical, mental, and social well-being, and not merely the absence of disease.

The World Health Organization has adopted health promotion and self-care as one of its major strategies in coming years for improving health throughout the world. In both developed and developing countries, appropriate self-care practiced in coordination with existing health-care systems has the potential for vastly improving health. In developing countries, in particular, there are strong reasons for continuing to encourage *traditional* self-care healing practices.

Health Promotion, Wellness, and Self-Care

While the concepts of disease prevention and health promotion are many centuries old, it is only in recent years that we have seen a dramatic resurgence of interest in prevention programs. The impact of life style, rate of life changes and our coping strategies are key to determining our health status at any time.

People are deeply interested in improving their health *at all ages.* Increased attention is now being given to the mind-body-spirit connection and the need for personal satisfaction and purpose in relation to total health.

To these ends, self-help groups have proliferated within the last few years. They have begun to meet almost every conceivable need including weight control, smoking cessation, stress control, alcohol cessation, spiritual growth, and help with bereavement and grief. It is estimated that at least several hundred different types of groups are active in the United States alone; most are expanding worldwide.

The self-care/self-help movement has had a dramatic impact—pointing to the need to take an active role in maintaining or improving personal health throughout the life span.

Our remedies oft in ourselves do lie. . .

— *Shakespeare*

States of health or disease are the expressions of the success or failure experienced by the organism in its efforts to respond adaptively to environmental challenge.

— *Rene Dubos*

. . . You don't get to choose how you're going to die, or when. You can only decide how you're going to live. . . Now.

— *Joan Baez*

Risk Reduction and Health Maintenance

Although heredity may increase risk for certain diseases, it is the interaction between our total environment and genetic background that determines our state of health. There is increasing evidence that health is strongly influenced by physical, social, economic, and family environments. Personal health habits play an enormously important role in the development as well as the prevention of many diseases and injuries. Most of today's serious health problems are related to personal lifestyle and health habits: excessive stress, smoking, drinking, poor nutrition, misuse of medications, and/or careless driving.

According to the Surgeon General, of the top ten causes of mortality in the United States at least seven could be substantially reduced if persons at risk adhered to the following five health habits:

- dietary improvement
- smoking cessation
- adequate exercise
- reduced alcohol intake
- hypertension control

Personal Choice Reflections:

Reflecting on the "stepping stones" of your life, what choices have you made along the way that shaped your health and well-being? What choices will you make today?

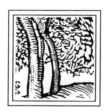

Pillars
of Health

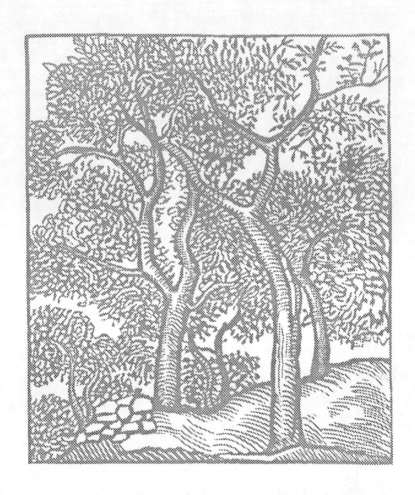

*In wilderness is the preservation
of the world.*   – *Thoreau*

Health signifies that one's life force is intact, and that one is sufficiently in harmony with the social, physical, and supernatural environment to enjoy what is positively valued in life.

— *Bantu African Thought*

▪ ▪ ▪

A vast potential capacity for change exists within every human being—regardless of age. The human mind is powerful beyond measure for disciplining the body and achieving wholeness. Personal health can be significantly improved through individual actions such as appropriate exercise, proper diet, and stress management–regarded as the three pillars of health promotion.

We are fast realizing that good health is not something that can be purchased at the corner pharmacy or from visiting a physician. Keeping the body and mind in optimal condition, well into our later years is largely a personal responsibility—a lifelong quest in which lifestyle and health habits make all the difference.

Given the mounting evidence that many major illnesses, including cardiovascular disease and some forms of cancer, are preventable, there is every reason to emphasize a strategy of health promotion and disease prevention throughout the life span. At each stage of life, different steps can be taken to maximize well-being. The individual plays an enormously important role in influencing the aging process. The ultimate goal, of course, is to live an independent and fulfilled life unencumbered by preventable illness.

Health-care providers in increasing numbers are promoting the idea of *wellness*. The goal of wellness is not just the absence of disease but the achievement of optimal health. It is a desirable condition for everyone, and it means tuning in to our own strengths and limitations early on, improving where possible, and avoiding what is harmful to our health.

■   ■   ■

Be not afraid of life. Believe that life is worth living, and your belief will help create the fact.
　　　　　　　　　　　　　　　　— W. James

Nutrition and Total Health

Probably no other area is as laden with controversy and myth as that of nutrition. No doubt this is due to the absolute relationship between food and the dynamic state of our health.

Nutritional status affects directly our mental, emotional, and physical well being. It is a cumulative process as well as an immediate one. With advancing age, our general state of health is determined to a great extent by the effects of dietary pattern over the years.

Nutritional requirements, food and drink preferences, and eating habits change throughout the life span. Each of these is influenced by a person's biological status as well as the physical and social environment.

There is considerable evidence that overeating is a serious problem at all ages. However, eating too little can be harmful as well. People who eat unbalanced diets may exhibit symptoms of nutrient deficiency including fatigue, irritability, anxiety, loss of recent memory, insomnia, lack of concentration, and even delusional states. All too often these correctable signs of malnutrition are attributed erroneously to "old age." Calcium, iron and B complex vitamins are the nutrients that have most often been found to be deficient in diets.

The role of various nutrients in maintaining good health must be emphasized throughout the life span, but it is never too late to adopt positive eating patterns. The importance of eating a balanced diet that provides adequate vitamins, minerals, protein, and complex carbohydrates must be emphasized. Such a diet is rich in fresh vegetables (especially leafy greens), fresh fruits, low-fat dairy products, legumes, fish, poultry, and whole grains. Water is also an essential nutrient, and care should be taken to ensure an adequate fluid intake at all times.

Learn to listen to your body . . . with an inner concentration . . .
to receive guidance as to when to exercise, when to rest and how to nourish yourself.

Basic Nutritional Guidelines

- Cut down on fat intake.

- Eat more complex carbohydrate and high-fiber foods, such as whole grain cereals, fruits, and vegetables.

- Reduce salt intake.

- Include in the daily diet foods rich in vitamins A and C.

- Include in the diet cruciferous vegetables such as cabbage, broccoli, Brussels sprouts, kohlrabi, and cauliflower.

- Limit or eliminate consumption of alcoholic beverages and caffeine.

- Limit consumption of salt-cured, smoked, and nitrite-cured foods.

Exercise and Health

Substantial evidence exists that exercise and movement are essential for health in all age groups. The power that movement has on mental and physical well-being is dramatic.

One of the unique features of the human body is that the more it is used—within reasonable limits—the better it works. There is ample evidence that exercise is a preventive action against a multitude of diseases. Not only do the lungs and circulatory system work better but the digestive system is stimulated, bowel function improves, and back weakness and pain are often prevented. Bones also benefit greatly from physical activity; exercises performed in a weight-bearing position, such as bicycling, jogging, or brisk walking, stimulate the formation of new bone. Combined with adequate calcium intake, exercise can also prevent abnormal bone loss and osteoporosis.

Regular exercise can retard changes that once were thought to be part of the aging process. In fact, a high proportion of the physical decline attributed to aging is actually the result of inactivity and poor nutrition. Regular physical activity can help the human body maintain, repair, and improve itself to an amazing degree.

Inactivity is a serious risk factor for coronary heart disease. Regular exercise, on the other hand, elevates levels of high-density lipoprotein (HDL), which is believed to slow or resist the build up of cholesterol in the arteries. Other risk factors such as stress, obesity and high blood pressure may be reduced by exercise as well.

People of all ages are showing interest in fitness, and this is by and large a very positive development. However, it is important to consider that there are individual-appropriate levels as well as age-appropriate levels of physical activity. Each person must learn to tune in to his or her own activity level and respond accordingly. Even those who are homebound can find ways of exercising more. Most older people—including those with illness or disabilities—can take part in moderate exercise programs. Many who are confined to wheelchairs can participate in a variety of exercise activities to improve their strength and sense of well-being.

Exercise cannot prevent the stresses of life but it can help us cope with them. Involvement in some kind of physical activity helps reduce mental fatigue and tension. Exercise is a terrific antidote for depression; it improves mood at the same time it enhances the ability to sleep restfully. Ample evidence exists that body activity can positively affect states of mind and quality of life. Walking and swimming are both excellent forms of exercise. The by-products of a good fitness program are increased self esteem, increased energy and a build up of lean body mass.

It is important to warm up the body for vigorous exercise by starting lightly with a continous rhythmical activity such as walking and gradually increasing the intensity until the pulse rate, breathing, and body temperature are elevated. Periods of vigorous activity should be alternated with periods of less stress. By gradually increasing the pace of activity, physical condition can be greatly improved.

Exercises that help burn up more calories than are ingested can help shed excess fat. Even for a specific problem area, spot exercise will not be more effective than overall conditioning activities because the body naturally loses fat from the areas of greatest excess. Exercise increases the calories the body uses every day, burns up excess fatty tissues while building up lean body mass so that vital active tissue is not lost, and keeps the percentage of body fat at the appropriate level.

While activity has to be sustained to obtain major benefits, the cumulative effect of exercises and activities carried on during a period of time counts. For example, every movement uses calories, but even though certain activities such as a short walk may not use many calories at a time, a number of short walks in the course of a day may together burn up quite a few calories. In the same manner, the benefits to organs, joints, and muscles add up little by little. So it is a good idea (at any age) to step up activity throughout the day in addition to following specifically planned periods of exercise.

Principles for Exercise:

- Determine a proper exercise regime.

- Start at a low, comfortable level of exercise and progress gradually.

- Know your limit and stay within it.

- Exercise regularly; a minimum of three times a week and a maximum of five times.

- Exercise at a rate within your capacity.

- Warm up and cool down before and after exercise.

Stress Management

Later life is sometimes accompanied by losses—loss of status, loss of social supports, or loss of loved ones. These circumstances, coupled with negative stereotypes of aging, can contribute to high levels of stress and tension.

Stress is a significant risk factor for heart disease and stroke and is known to be a contributor to nearly all chronic illness. Consequently, reducing or managing excessive stress is essential for improving health and for managing as well as preventing chronic disease.

The term *stress* is often used loosely. People tend to use stress to describe both external factors and physical reactions.

In recent years, much emphasis has been placed on the study of stress; however, it was Hans Selye who provided the initial understanding. How does stress affect us? According to Selye there are three stages:

1. Alarm

This first stage is the mobilization of the body's defenses. Messages from the nervous system reach the hypothalamus gland, which notifies the pituitary gland and the adrenal gland. The pituitary–adrenal system pumps hormones into the bloodstream. The hormones have the effect of speeding the heart rate, increasing respiration, and stopping digestive activity.

2. *Resistance and Adaptation*

In this stage the invader is fought off or some adjustment is made. If tired, one sleeps. If hungry, one eats. If a large number of microbes are in a wound, inflammation promotes healing. This defense system works so well that most of the time we are unaware of it. We are all regularly confronted by environmental challenges and, for the most part, we adapt and resist illness. However, if the stress is severe and prolonged, a state of exhaustion can occur.

3. *Exhaustion*

The physical body cannot be under severe stress all the time, and there is evidence that numerous health problems are stress induced — colds, allergies, asthma, headaches, ulcers, colitis, heart disease, arthritis, and sundry other illnesses.

*The tragedy of life is not death, but
what we let die within us while we live.*

– Norman Cousins

■　　■　　■

There is now general agreement regarding the importance of the role stress plays in disease. Stress can be defined as a complex problem involving physiological, psychological, and social phenomena interacting at various levels.

Selye distinguishes between eustress and distress, emphasizing that stress can be either good or bad, helpful or hurtful. He advises:

Don't try to avoid stress but master it and channel it into the form of eustress rather than distress; find the occupation or activity that is pleasant for you and that you are good at. If you are poor at something and continuously humiliated by failure, obviously that is negative. On the other hand, if you find purposeful activity that enhances your self-esteem and sense of mastery, that is excellent.

Learn to distinguish when to submit and when to

fight—knowing this will preserve and lengthen your life. Avoid the self-destructive distress of failure, frustration and hatred. Seek the pleasant stress of fulfillment and victory.

Don't feel guilty about your natural egotism. Recognize that "altruistic egotism"—helping others in order to gain their love, respect, good-will and trust—gives you a sense of security and self-esteem to cushion against the many frustrations and hurts of life.

Techniques of relaxation to reduce stress are multiple and varied. There are the familiar, simple, old-fashioned techniques: leaving a tense situation to take a brisk walk; relaxing in a hot tub; having someone gently massage your neck or back muscles; getting rid of pent-up emotion or anger through vigorous physical activity. Other highly effective methods of stress reduction include meditation, deep breathing, and visualization—preventive imagery.

Meditation

Most people carry on numerous internal dialogues throughout the day. Self-talk is an integral part of everyone's makeup. Meditation is a form of self-listening. It is a way of calming the mind and body, letting in healing energy, and getting in touch with the inner self.

By quieting the mind through meditation, blood pressure can be lowered, heart rate decreased, less oxygen used, and alpha (brain) waves increased.

Meditation is a calm silencing of the mind that in turn helps to develop increased mental clarity. Over time a clear, more comprehensive understanding of self—a sense of wholeness and equanimity occurs.

■　　■　　■

Everything that is — is within.　　*–Anon*

■　　■　　■

Let retrospectives make their peace in your heart.　　*– Gerimar*

Breathing

Learning to breathe deeply and experience relaxation can be very satisfying and is a vital part of managing stress at any age. To enhance your sense of well-being:

- Breathe deeply by dropping the diaphragm so that the abdomen is pushed out. Breathe in through the nose and out through the mouth.

- Breathe deeply with vibrating sounds or words repeated over and over with the exhalation.

- For relaxation and falling asleep, breathe into the abdomen and continue to inhale deeply and slowly. Breathe out very slowly and pause before breathing in again. Keep thinking about your breathing. It may help to keep a slow rhythm if you visualize a gull flying, moonlight on the ocean, waves slowly rising and falling, or waves breaking on the beach with the water slowly sinking into the sand.

- For pain or tension at any place in your body, as you breathe focus your attention on that spot and imagine your breath going out through that place and carrying the pain or stiffness with it.

After you have done any of the breathing exercises, just continue this quiet process of completely filling and emptying the lungs. Close your eyes and concentrate on your breathing to the exclusion of everything else. Feel everything you can about breathing. Relax your face and your mind, and just visualize the energy flowing in and out of your body. Feel this subtle energy of breath that everything in life depends upon. Jot down your thoughts and feelings at this moment in the space below.

Preventive Imagery

Some self-care practices require considerable investments of time, effort, and planning; others are relatively simple, such as the use of preventive imagery. Preventive imagery involves picturing what is happening inside the body and noting any blockages and areas of tension or tightness.

Imagery and creative visualization have a long and varied history in healing traditions. Most uses of imagery in the self-care movement involve techniques of relaxation, pain control, and autonomic self-regulation.

The human imagination is perhaps one of the most useful therapeutic tools available to us to care for ourselves. The techniques of creative visualization are myriad; their essence is to visualize the self whole and well—as one wishes to be—and to focus on that potential reality. Not only can this process help identify goals to work toward but it can also mobilize us to pursue those goals.

The positive results that have been demonstrated suggest that imagery-visualization leads to an enhancement of the immune system. The human (body/mind/spirit) is indeed capable of caring for itself, and this realization has a far-reaching impact.

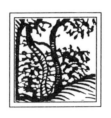

Integrating
Mind-Body-Spirit

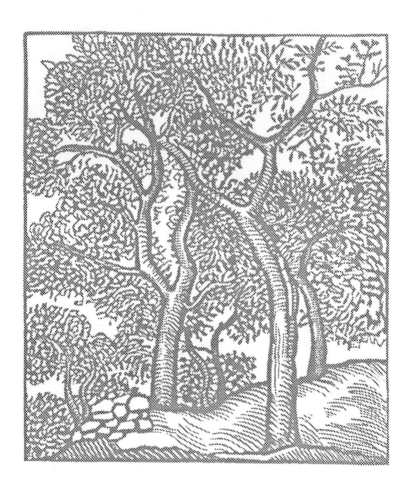

*There is nothing stronger in the world
than gentleness.* — Han Suyin

To everything there is a season...and a time to every purpose under the heavens.

— *Ecclesiastes*

The Holistic Approach to Health

The holistic perspective sees physical, mental, spiritual, and emotional states as totally interrelated with one another and with the environment.

Holistic health can be described as a process that is at once dynamic and evolving. The unity of *body*, *mind* and *spirit* is a view commonly accepted by most of the world's people; the separation of these three parts of the whole person seems to be unique to Western civilization in modern times. Increasingly, however, we are gaining a keen awareness of the need to return to the integrated holistic picture of humankind.

Wellness is a concept, a value, a lifestyle, and a process. The word *wellness*, like the word *health*, means different things to different individuals. A most commonly accepted definition encompasses feeling sufficiently good about oneself to take stock of one's own life and to intervene and nourish the *whole self* as necessary.

Health care is definitely turning in the direction of self-care and wellness. Trend analysts foresee a focus on individual responsibility for disease prevention and health promotion in the coming decades. Following are some aspects of that future view:

- Belief that physical disease is a symptom of some underlying emotional, mental, social, psychological or spiritual pathology will be prevalent.

- Emphasis on competition and survival of the fittest will be seen as pathology that breaks down the body's ability to maintain equilibrium.

- There will be few limits to an individual's responsibilities for his or her own health. Children will be taught techniques to encourage their bodies to adapt naturally to overcome illness.

- There will be substantial reliance on community-based healers such as educators, osteopaths, acupuncturists, massage therapists, and ethnic or traditional practitioners.

- Dying will be viewed as an opportunity for spiritual growth; few terminally ill people will be kept alive by high technology.

- Health care will focus on the integration of mind-body-spirit. Research will concentrate on determining what constitutes wellness and why some people are extraordinarily well — even in stressful situations.

- There will be greater respect for the environment; it will be understood that individual wellness and social wellness cannot be separated.

- People will increasingly pursue spiritual growth as a means toward achieving wholeness and health.

- Health care providers and consumers alike will actively promote and seek inner serenity through self-help groups and individual introspection and reflection.

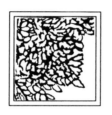

Serenity
Affirmations
and
Joyful Aging

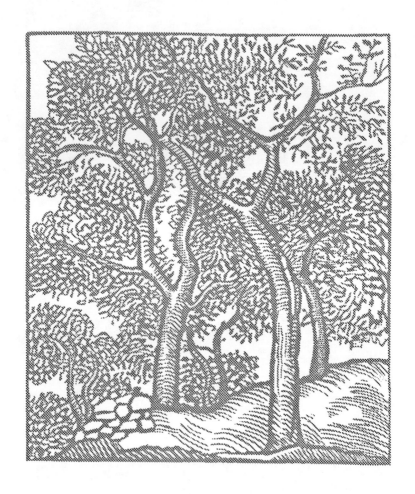

Be able to be alone . . . lose not the advantage of solitude. — T. Browne

Serenity

Grant me the serenity to accept the things I cannot change, the courage to change the things I can, and the wisdom to know the difference.

– R. Niebuhr

As the shift to wellness and self-care takes place, more and more people are achieving a sense of wholeness and serenity through the use of *affirmations.* An affirmation is a positive thought or idea that you consciously focus on in order to produce a desired result. It is a simple yet profound technique that often brings about dramatic results — transforming attitudes and creating inner peace.

To receive a profound sense of peace and purpose: Begin each day — for 28 days — by reading aloud the above "Serenity" poem.

The following *Serenity Affirmations* are being used by many in the process of healing past hurts and relationships and growing into *wholeness*.

Select one Serenity Affirmation each day for 28 days and repeat it silently throughout the day . . . You may choose to create your own Serenity Affirmations for the last 7 days of the 28 day cycle, or you may wish to repeat those that are most meaningful to you.

Make a promise to yourself each day and write it next to your Serenity Affirmation for the day. Reflect upon the increasing sense of peace and purpose that you are experiencing, and jot down your thoughts and feelings at the end of each day.

1. Serenity is . . .
living one day at a time.
Just for today I

_____

_____

2. Serenity is . . .
trusting in the now.
Just for today I

_____

3. Serenity is . . .
being open and willing to change.

Just for today I

_____

_____

4. Serenity is . . .
remembering to be grateful.

Just for today I

_____

_____

5. Serenity is . . .
taking one step at a time.

Just for today I

_____

_____

6. Serenity is . . .
following my inner voice.

Just for today I

_____

_____

7. Serenity is . . .
treating myself gently.

Just for today I

_____

_____

8. Serenity is . . .
letting go of all resentment.

Just for today I

_____

_____

9. Serenity is . . .
accepting each day.

Just for today I

_____

_____

10. Serenity is . . .
surrendering and trusting.

Just for today I

_____

_____

11. Serenity is . . .
living fully and feeling protected.

Just for today I

_____

_____

12. Serenity is . . .
acknowledging joy and beauty in my life.

Just for today I

_____

_____

13. Serenity is . . .
living in harmony with the Universe.

Just for today I

_____

_____

14. *Serenity is . . .*
keeping it simple.

Just for today I

_____

_____

15. *Serenity is . . .*
being honest with myself.

Just for today I

_____

_____

16. *Serenity is . . .*
forgiving the past.

Just for today I

_____

_____

17. *Serenity is . . .*
respecting myself.

Just for today I

_____

_____

18. *Serenity is . . .*
       recognizing my self-worth.
    Just for today I

    _____

    _____

19. *Serenity is . . .*
       listening deep within myself.
    Just for today I

    _____

    _____

20. *Serenity is . . .*
       letting the mystery of life
       unfold within me.
    Just for today I

    _____

    _____

21. *Serenity is . . .*
       keeping a rainbow in my heart.
    Just for today I

    _____

22. *Serenity is . . .*

_____

Just for today I

_____

_____

23. *Serenity is . . .*

_____

Just for today I

_____

_____

24. *Serenity is . . .*

_____

Just for today I

_____

_____

25. *Serenity is . . .*

_____

Just for today I

_____

_____

26. Serenity is . . .

Just for today I

27. Serenity is . . .

Just for today I

28. Serenity is . . .

Just for today I

Keep dreaming . . .
  Keep believing . . .
    Keep a rainbow in your heart.

Look to this Day

Look to this day,
For it is life,
The very life of life.
In its brief course lie all
The realities and truths of existence,
The joy of growth,
The splendor of action,
The glory of power —
For yesterday is but a dream
And tomorrow is only a vision.
But today, well lived,
Makes every yesterday a memory of
happiness
And every tomorrow a vision of hope.
Look well, therefore, to this day.

— Sanskrit Proverb

Thoughts and Affirmations

Thoughts can heal the body because thoughts created its need to be healed.

— Anon

We create all our tomorrows by what we dream today.

We grow in time to trust the future for our answers.

—Ruth Benedict

Dreams are the touchstones of our character.

— Thoreau

Faith is the bird that sings when the dawn is still dark.   – Tagore

Happiness is the meaning and purpose of life, the whole aim and end of human existence.   – Aristotle

Even a happy life cannot be without a measure of darkness . . . the word "happiness" would lose its meaning if it were not balanced by sadness.

– Carl Jung

Happiness is not a state to arrive at but a manner of traveling.

– Margaret Lee Runbeck

To live means sharing one another's space, dreams, sorrows; contributing our ears to hear, our eyes to see, our arms to hold, our hearts to love.

– Paul Tillich

■　　■　　■

The purpose of life is to leave the world a little better for having lived.

– Helen Green Ansley

■　　■　　■

The good life is a process, not a state of being. It is a direction, not a destination.

– Carl Rogers

■　　■　　■

Live each day as if your life had just begun.

– Goethe

One is never so happy as when the mind, the senses, and the heart are all working harmoniously together.

— *Seneca*

* * *

There are many paths to wisdom and to the heart; when one presents itself — if it fits — follow it; if not — move on. Another will emerge. Trust the process.

—Gerimar

* * *

Do not follow where the path may lead. Go, instead, where there is no path and leave a trail.

— *Anon*

Whatever you can do,
Or dream you can,
Begin it.
Boldness has genius,
power and magic in it.
Begin it now.

– Goethe

* * *

A thousand mile journey begins with
a single step. *– Lao Tse*

* * *

Life without idealism is empty
indeed. We must have hope . . .

– Pearl Buck

Old age and the wear of time teach many things. — Sophocles

In the midst of winter, I finally learned that there was in me an Invincible Summer. — Camus

Life goes not backward nor tarries with yesterday. — Gibran

Birds sing after a storm; why shouldn't people feel as free to delight in whatever remains to them?

— Rose Fitzgerald Kennedy

Aging is the process of weaving the tapestry of our lives . . . through maturity and progress. —Gerimar

Search for meaning is the primary motivation in life. – Viktor Frankl

*Everyone has a message.
Our lives are our message.*
—Ghandi

The surest way to live with honor in the world is to be in reality what we would appear to be.
– Socrates

Old age, to the unlearned, is winter; to the learned it is harvest time.

—*Yiddish Proverb*

■　　■　　■

Old age, especially an honored old age, has so great authority, that this is of more value than all the pleasure of youth.　　—*Cicero*

■　　■　　■

Let us cherish and love old age; for it is full of pleasure, if one knows how to use it.　　—*Seneca*

■　　■　　■

One cannot have wisdom without living life.　　—*Dorothy McCall*

In the autumn of your life, let every leaf be shining gold.

— Ann M. Gartrell

■   ■   ■

Grow old with me, the best is yet to be, the last of life for which the first was made . . . — Robert Browning

■   ■   ■

Aging is a spiritual journey with challenges and opportunities to grow all along the way. — Gerimar

■   ■   ■

In quietness and confidence shall be your strength. — Isaiah

Be true to the highest within your soul.
                                    —R.W. Trine

Intelligence highly awakened is intuition.
                                    — Krishnamurti

It doesn't happen all at once . . . You become . . . it takes a long time.
                                    — Margery Williams

This we know, the earth does not belong to us, we belong to the earth. This we know, all things are connected, like the blood which unites one family. All things are connected.
                                    — Chief Seattle

We cannot discover new oceans until we have courage to lose sight of the shore. — *Anon*

■   ■   ■

There are believers in life and the bounty of life, and their coffer is never empty. — *Gibran*

■   ■   ■

The best and most beautiful things in the world cannot be seen or even touched — they must be felt with the heart. — *Helen Keller*

■   ■   ■

On wings of love hearts can travel free.

Success

To laugh often and much;
To win the respect of intelligent people
and the affection of children;
To earn the appreciation of honest
critics and endure the betrayal of
false friends;
To appreciate beauty, to find the best
in others;
To leave the world a bit better,
whether by a healthy child, a garden
patch or a redeemed social condition;
To know even one life has breathed
easier because you have lived.
This is to have succeeded.

—Emerson

If we love beauty,
If we love health,
If we love to create joy,
We become what we love.

■   ■   ■

This world is not conclusion;
A sequel stands beyond,
Invisible, as music,
But positive, as sound.

—Emily Dickinson

■   ■   ■

We have loved the stars too fondly to
be fearful of the night.   *– Anon*

References

Ansley, Helen Green. *Life's Finishing School.* Sausalito, CA: Institute of Noetic Sciences.

Benson, Herbert. *The Mind/Body Effect.* New York: Simon and Schuster.

Benson, Herbert and Miriam Klipper. *The Relaxation Response.* New York: Avon Books.

Borysenko, Joan. *Minding the Body, Mending the Mind.* New York; Bantam Books.

Burdman, Geri Marr. *Healthful Aging.* Englewood Cliffs, NJ: Prentice-Hall, Inc.

Butler, Robert and M. I. Lewis. *Aging and Mental Health.* St. Louis: C.V. Mosby Co.

Chopra, Deepak. *Quantum Healing.* New York: Bantam Books.

Comfort, Alex, *A Good Age,* New York: Crown.

Council of Life Insurance. *Trend Analysis Program Reports.* Washington, D.C.

Cousins, Norman. *Anatomy of an Illness.* New York: W.W. Norton.

Cousins, Norman. *Head First : The Biology of Hope.* New York: E.P. Dutton.

Dychtwald, Ken. *Age Wave.* Los Angeles: Jeremy P. Tarcher.

DeVries, Herbert A. and D. Holes. *Fitness After Fifty.* New York: McGraw Hill.

Erikson, Erik. *Childhood and Society.* New York: W.W. Norton & Co., Inc.

Erikson, Joan M. *Wisdom and the Senses.* New York: W.W. Norton & Co., Inc.

Frankl, Viktor. *Man's Search for Meaning*. Boston: Beacon Press.

Fries, James and L. Crapo. *Vitality and Aging*. San Francisco: W.H. Freeman & Co.

Gawain, Shakti. *Creative Visualization*. New York: Bantam Books.

Goble , Frank G. *The Third Force. The Psychology of Abraham Maslow*. New York: Grossman.

Harmon, Willis. *Higher Creativity*. Los Angeles: Jeremy P. Tarcher.

LeShan, Lawrence. *How to Meditate*. New York: Bantam Books.

Matthews-Simonton, Stephanie, O. Carl Simonton, and James L. Creighton. *Getting Well Again*. New York: Bantam Books.

Nouwen, Henri and W.J. Gaffney. *Aging and Fulfillment of Life,* Garden City, New York: Image Books.

Pelletier, Kenneth. *Longevity: Fulfilling our Biological Potential*. New York: Dell Books.

Pelletier, Kenneth. *Mind as Healer, Mind as Slayer: A Holistic Approach to Preventing Stress Disorders*. New York: Delta.

Seyle, Hans. *The Stress of Life*. New York: McGraw Hill.

Seigel, Bernie. *Love, Medicine and Miracles*. New York: Harper & Row.

Seigel, Bernie. *Peace, Love, and Healing*. New York: Harper & Row.

Weil, Andrew. *Health and Healing: Understanding Conventional and Alternative Medicine*. Boston: Houghton Mifflin.

About the author . . .

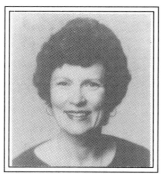

Geri Marr Burdman, Ph.D., R.N., is a gerontologist, health educator, rehabilitation counselor and international health specialist. She has conducted study tours and has served as a consultant in many parts of the world including Asia, Australia, Africa, Latin America, and the Caribbean.

As an international consultant and lecturer on Health Promotion and Aging, Dr. Marr Burdman offers a unique interdisciplinary perspective on aging, relating biological, psychological, and sociological phenomena to the integration of mind-body-spirit. Her focus throughout is on preserving the quality of life into the later years.

Geri is deeply committed to sharing her perceptions of the oneness of humankind and the common thread that connects us all. Through personal growth and aging classes, workshops and retreats, she assists participants to go into the quiet place within themselves, to connect more deeply with nature and to find serenity and inner peace.

For information on publications and workshops:

GERIMAR PUBLICATIONS
P.O. Box 357
Mercer Island, WA 98040 USA
(206) 232-7029